POLYMYALGIA TICA

DIET

Relief Through Food - A Personalized Diet Guide for Polymyalgia Rheumatic

SELENA LEONARD

Copyright© 2024 [Selena Leonard]

All rights reserved. Unauthorized reproduction or distribution of this work is strictly prohibited or transmitted in any form or by any means, including photocopying, recording, or other electronic or methods, without the prior written permission of the publisher, except in the case of brief quotations embodied in critical articles and reviews.

Table of Contents

INTRODUCTION 9

EMBRACING FOOD AS A POWERFUL ALLY IN MANAGING POLYMYALGIA RHEUMATICA 9

    Understanding Polymyalgia Rheumatica: 9

CHAPTER 1 13

ESSENTIAL ANTI-INFLAMMATORY INGREDIENTS - BUILDING THE FOUNDATION OF YOUR PMR DIET 13

    Focus on Omega-3 Fatty Acids: Exploring the Benefits of Fatty Fish (Salmon): 13

    The Power of Plants: Utilizing Fruits, Vegetables, and Leafy Greens (Spinach, Tomatoes, Berry): 14

    The Mighty Mediterranean: Embracing Olive Oil for its Anti-inflammatory Properties: 16

CHAPTER 2 19

NAVIGATING THE FOOD LANDSCAPE: FOODS TO LIMIT OR AVOID 19

    Pro-Inflammatory Culprits: Refined Carbohydrates, Sugary Drinks, and Processed Foods: 19

CHAPTER 3 23

BUILDING A PERSONALIZED MEAL PLAN - YOUR ROADMAP TO DELICIOUS RELIEF 23

    Portion Control and Mindful Eating: 25

    Sample Meal Plans for Different Dietary Needs: 25

    Sample Meal Plan (Vegetarian): 26

    Sample Meal Plan (Gluten-Free): 26

CHAPTER 4 29

STARTING YOUR DAY RIGHT - FUELING YOUR BODY FOR AN ACTIVE MORNING WITH PMR 29

    Omega-3 Powerhouse - Scrambled Eggs with Smoked Salmon and Spinach 29

    Berrylicious Smoothie - Packed with Antioxidants and Chia Seeds for Fiber 31

CHAPTER 5 35

LIGHT AND NOURISHING LUNCHES - POWERING THROUGH YOUR AFTERNOON WITH PMR 35

    Mediterranean Feast - Salmon Salad with Chopped Vegetables and Olive Oil Dressing 35

    Leafy Green Goodness - Spinach Salad with Walnuts, Berries, and Goat Cheese (modify cheese if needed) 38

Anti-Inflammatory Wrap - Turkey and Veggie Wrap with Whole-Wheat Tortilla 40

CHAPTER 6 45

FLAVORFUL AND SATISFYING DINNERS - NOURISHING YOUR BODY FOR A RESTFUL NIGHT WITH PMR 45

One-Pan Wonder - Roasted Salmon with Vegetables and Herbs 45

Veggie Power Bowl - Quinoa Bowl with Roasted Vegetables and Tahini Dressing 48

Anti-Inflammatory Pasta Delight - Whole-Wheat Pasta with Shrimp and Spinach Pesto 50

CHAPTER 7 55

SMART SNACKING FOR SUSTAINED ENERGY - POWERING THROUGH YOUR DAY WITH PMR 55

Trail Mix Powerhouse - Homemade Trail Mix with Nuts, Seeds, and Dried Fruit (modify based on tolerated ingredients) 55

Energy Bites - Antioxidant-Rich Energy Bites with Dates, Nuts, and Seeds 57

CHAPTER 8 63

ADDITIONAL TIPS FOR MANAGING POLYMYALGIA RHEUMATICA - OPTIMIZING YOUR WELL-BEING BEYOND DIET 63

    1. Importance of Exercise and Movement: 63

    2. Prioritizing Sleep and Relaxation Techniques 64

    3. Importance of Hydration: 65

    4. The Mind-Body Connection: Stress Management and Emotional Wellbeing: 66

CHAPTER 9 69

BUILDING A SUPPORT SYSTEM - A NETWORK FOR STRENGTH AND SHARED EXPERIENCES WITH PMR 69

    1. Communicating with Your Doctor and Healthcare Team: 69

    2. The Power of Support Groups and Online Communities . 70

CHAPTER 10 73

A LOOK TO THE FUTURE: MAINTAINING A POSITIVE OUTLOOK WITH PMR 73

    1. The Power of Positive Thinking 73

    2. Effective Stress Management 74

    3. Embracing a Proactive Approach: 76

BONUS CHAPTER 79

BONUS RECIPES FOR POLYMYALGIA RHEUMATIC DIET 79

Flavorful and Satisfying Dinners - Nourishing Your Body for a Restful Night with PMR 79

One-Pan Wonder - Roasted Salmon with Spinach and Tomatoes 79

Protein Power Bowl - Quinoa with Roasted Vegetables and Almonds 81

Sheet Pan Frittata with Spinach and Cherry Tomatoes 83

Spiced Salmon with Berry Salsa 85

One-Pan Lemon Garlic Shrimp with Leafy Greens 87

Vegetarian Chili with Quinoa and Black Beans 89

Creamy Spinach and Mushroom Pasta with Walnuts 91

Baked Eggs with Frittata Toppings 93

Salmon Burgers with Almond Flour Buns 95

Chicken Stir-Fry with Vegetables and Brown Rice 98

Lentil Soup with Leafy Greens and Lemon 101

Vegetarian Stuffed Peppers 103

Tofu Scramble with Spinach and Tomatoes 105

Chicken and Vegetable Curry with Coconut Milk 107

One-Pan Roasted Chicken with Root Vegetables............... 109

Turkey Burgers with Sweet Potato Fries 111

Lentil and Vegetable Shepherd's Pie 114

Chicken and Quinoa Stuffed Peppers 114

Salmon with Roasted Vegetables and Lemon Dill Sauce... 116

CONCLUSION 119

INTRODUCTION

EMBRACING FOOD AS A POWERFUL ALLY IN MANAGING POLYMYALGIA RHEUMATICA

Have you been diagnosed with Polymyalgia Rheumatica (PMR)? If so, you're likely experiencing a range of symptoms like stiffness, pain, and fatigue that can significantly impact your daily life. While there's no cure for PMR, there are effective treatment options available, and you can play a proactive role in managing your symptoms. This book introduces a powerful tool in your PMR management toolbox: **food**.

Understanding Polymyalgia Rheumatica:

PMR is an autoimmune inflammatory condition primarily affecting the muscles around your shoulders, hips, and upper body. The exact cause remains unknown, but it's believed that the body's immune system mistakenly attacks healthy tissues, leading to inflammation and pain. This inflammation can also contribute to fatigue, a common symptom of PMR.

The Anti-Inflammatory Power of Food:

While medication plays a crucial role in managing PMR, research suggests that diet can also be a powerful ally. Certain foods possess natural anti-inflammatory properties, meaning they can help reduce inflammation throughout the body, potentially easing PMR symptoms like stiffness and pain.

This book delves into the science behind these anti-inflammatory foods and explores how incorporating them into your diet can support your overall well-being. We'll discuss essential ingredients like omega-3 fatty acids found in fatty fish, the benefits of fruits, vegetables, and leafy greens, and the role of healthy fats like those found in nuts and seeds.

Personalized Approach to Your Polymyalgia Rheumatica Diet:

We understand that everyone's body and dietary needs are unique. This book won't prescribe a one-size-fits-all approach. Instead, we'll guide you through the process of creating a personalized PMR diet plan that caters to your preferences and any existing dietary restrictions.

By learning about anti-inflammatory foods, understanding what foods might exacerbate symptoms, and creating a balanced meal plan, you can harness the power of food to feel better and manage your PMR effectively. Let's embark on this journey together and explore how delicious and nutritious meals can become a cornerstone of your well-being.

PART 1: BUILDING YOUR FOUNDATION

CHAPTER 1

ESSENTIAL ANTI-INFLAMMATORY INGREDIENTS - BUILDING THE FOUNDATION OF YOUR PMR DIET

Polymyalgia Rheumatica (PMR) can significantly impact your daily life with symptoms like stiffness, pain, and fatigue. This chapter introduces you to the key players in your PMR dietary toolbox: **anti-inflammatory foods**. By incorporating these ingredients into your meals, you can potentially reduce inflammation, alleviate PMR symptoms, and support your overall well-being. Let's explore some of the most powerful anti-inflammatory ingredients you'll encounter throughout this book:

Focus on Omega-3 Fatty Acids: Exploring the Benefits of Fatty Fish (Salmon):

- **The Science Behind Omega-3s:** Fatty fish like salmon, mackerel, sardines, and herring are rich in omega-3 fatty acids, particularly EPA and DHA. These essential fats possess potent anti-inflammatory properties. Research suggests that omega-3s can help reduce inflammatory markers in the body, potentially easing pain and stiffness associated with PMR.

- **Beyond Inflammation:** Omega-3s offer additional benefits beyond their anti-inflammatory effects. They play a crucial role in brain health, supporting cognitive function and memory. Omega-3s also contribute to heart health by lowering bad cholesterol (LDL) and reducing the risk of blood clots.

- **Delicious and Easy Incorporation:** Fatty fish is a versatile ingredient that can be enjoyed in various ways. Bake, broil, or grill salmon for a quick and healthy meal. Salmon can also be incorporated into salads, sandwiches, or pasta dishes. Aim to include at least two servings of fatty fish per week in your PMR diet plan.

The Power of Plants: Utilizing Fruits, Vegetables, and Leafy Greens (Spinach, Tomatoes, Berry):

1. **A Rainbow of Antioxidants:** Fruits, vegetables, and leafy greens are packed with antioxidants, which help combat free radicals in the body. Free radicals contribute to

inflammation, and antioxidants can help neutralize them, potentially reducing overall inflammation and easing PMR symptoms.

2. **Fiber Powerhouse:** Many fruits and vegetables are rich in fiber, which promotes gut health and aids in digestion. A healthy gut microbiome is linked to reduced inflammation throughout the body.

3. **Vitamins and Minerals:** Fruits and vegetables provide essential vitamins and minerals that support overall health and well-being. Vitamin C, for example, is a powerful antioxidant, and vitamin D plays a role in immune function.

4. **Variety is Key:** Explore the vibrant world of fruits, vegetables, and leafy greens! Incorporate a variety of colors on your plate to ensure you're getting a diverse range of antioxidants and nutrients. Spinach, tomatoes, and berries are just a few examples, but don't be afraid to experiment with different options. Aim for at least five servings of fruits and vegetables daily.

Healthy Fats for You: Understanding the Role of Nuts and Seeds (Walnuts, Almonds):

1. **Not All Fats are Created Equal:** While some fats can contribute to inflammation, others offer significant health

benefits. Nuts and seeds are a great source of healthy fats, including monounsaturated and polyunsaturated fats. These fats have been shown to have anti-inflammatory properties.

2. **Beyond Inflammation:** Nuts and seeds are nutritional powerhouses. They are a good source of protein, fiber, vitamins, and minerals. These nutrients contribute to overall health and support a strong immune system.

3. **Snacking Smart:** Nuts and seeds are a convenient and portable snack option. They are also a great way to add healthy fats and protein to your meals. Choose raw or dry-roasted nuts and seeds for the most health benefits. Aim for a moderate handful (around 1 ounce) per day.

4. **Variety is Key:** Explore different types of nuts and seeds like walnuts, almonds, flaxseeds, and chia seeds. Each variety offers a unique nutritional profile.

The Mighty Mediterranean: Embracing Olive Oil for its Anti-inflammatory Properties:

- **Liquid Gold:** Olive oil, a staple of the Mediterranean diet, has been praised for its health benefits for centuries. Extra virgin olive oil is rich in monounsaturated fats, particularly oleic acid, which possesses anti-inflammatory properties.

- **Beyond Inflammation:** Olive oil is a good source of antioxidants that can help protect against heart disease and certain cancers. It also contributes to healthy blood sugar control.
- **Cooking with Confidence:** Olive oil is a versatile cooking oil with a high smoke point, making it suitable for various cooking methods like sauteing, roasting, and dressing salads. Choose extra virgin olive oil for its superior flavor and health benefits.
- **Drizzle, Don't Drench:** While olive oil is a healthy fat, it's still high in calories. Use it moderately. A drizzle is enough to add flavor and reap the benefits without

CHAPTER 2

NAVIGATING THE FOOD LANDSCAPE: FOODS TO LIMIT OR AVOID

While Chapter 1 focused on the anti-inflammatory heroes of your PMR diet, this chapter explores the foods that might hinder your progress. Understanding which foods can potentially exacerbate inflammation is key to creating an effective PMR dietary plan.

Pro-Inflammatory Culprits: Refined Carbohydrates, Sugary Drinks, and Processed Foods:

The Refined Carbohydrate Conundrum: Refined carbohydrates, found in white bread, pastries, sugary cereals, and white rice, can cause blood sugar spikes. These spikes can trigger inflammatory responses in the body, potentially worsening PMR symptoms like stiffness and pain.

- **Sugary Drinks: A Double Whammy:** Sugary drinks like soda, sweetened juices, and sports drinks are loaded with refined sugar. Sugar not only contributes to blood sugar spikes but also feeds unhealthy gut bacteria, potentially increasing inflammation.

- **Processed Food Peril:** Processed foods are often high in unhealthy fats, refined carbohydrates, added sugar, and sodium. These ingredients can all contribute to inflammation and should be limited in a PMR diet. Processed foods are also typically low in essential nutrients that support overall well-being.

- **Making Smarter Choices:** Opt for whole grains like brown rice, quinoa, and whole-wheat bread instead of refined carbohydrates. Quench your thirst with water, unsweetened tea, or black coffee. Limit processed foods and opt for fresh, whole ingredients whenever possible.

Understanding Red Meat and Saturated Fats:

- **Saturated Fat and Inflammation:** While some healthy fats play a vital role in your PMR diet, saturated fats found in red meat (beef, lamb, pork) can contribute to inflammation. Excessive consumption of red meat has been linked to increased levels of inflammatory markers in the body.

- **Focus on Lean Cuts and Moderation:** If you enjoy red meat, choose lean cuts and limit your intake. Aim for no more than a few servings per week.

- **Alternative Protein Sources:** Explore other protein sources like fatty fish, chicken, turkey, beans, lentils, and tofu. These options provide protein without the saturated fat content often found in red meat.

Moderation is Key: Navigating Dairy Products:

- **The Dairy Debate:** The impact of dairy products on inflammation can vary depending on the individual. Some people with PMR find that dairy consumption worsens their symptoms, while others tolerate it well.

- **Listen to Your Body:** Pay close attention to how you feel after consuming dairy products. If you experience increased stiffness, pain, or fatigue, it might be beneficial to limit or eliminate dairy from your diet.

- **Dairy Alternatives:** If you choose to limit dairy, explore lactose-free options or plant-based alternatives like almond milk, soy milk, and coconut milk. These alternatives provide calcium and other nutrients found in dairy without the lactose, which can be problematic for some people.

CHAPTER 3

BUILDING A PERSONALIZED MEAL PLAN - YOUR ROADMAP TO DELICIOUS RELIEF

Now that you've explored the power of anti-inflammatory foods and gained insights into potentially inflammatory ingredients, it's time to translate this knowledge into action! This chapter empowers you to create a personalized meal plan that caters to your unique needs, preferences, and dietary restrictions.

Assessing Your Needs and Preferences:

1. **Understanding Your Body:** Before diving into meal planning, take a moment to reflect on your body's needs and preferences. Consider any existing dietary restrictions you might have, such as allergies or intolerances.
2. **Activity Level:** Are you physically active? A higher activity level might require adjustments to your calorie intake to ensure you're fueling your body adequately.

3. **Taste Preferences:** What kind of food do you enjoy? A successful meal plan is one you'll stick to, so consider incorporating flavors and cuisines you find appealing.
4. **Cooking Skills and Time Constraints:** Be realistic about your cooking skills and time available for meal preparation. If you're short on time, explore simple recipes or consider meal prepping on weekends.

Creating a Balanced Plate:

Your personalized PMR diet plan should revolve around the concept of a balanced plate. Imagine your plate divided into sections:

1. **Half Your Plate:** Fill half your plate with a variety of non-starchy vegetables like spinach, tomatoes, broccoli, peppers, and leafy greens. These nutrient-rich vegetables provide essential vitamins, minerals, and fiber, promoting gut health and potentially reducing inflammation.
2. **One Quarter Protein Powerhouse:** Allocate a quarter of your plate to lean protein sources like fatty fish (salmon, tuna), chicken, turkey, beans, lentils, or tofu. Protein is essential for building and repairing tissues, supporting a healthy immune system, and promoting satiety.

3. **One Quarter Whole Grains or Healthy Complex Carbs:** The remaining quarter of your plate can be filled with whole grains like brown rice, quinoa, whole-wheat pasta, or sweet potato. These complex carbohydrates provide sustained energy without causing significant blood sugar spikes.

Portion Control and Mindful Eating:

- **Mindful Matters:** Mindful eating is about paying attention to your body's hunger and fullness cues. Eat slowly, savor your food, and avoid distractions while eating. This allows you to recognize satiety and prevent overeating.
- **Portion Perfection:** Use measuring cups, spoons, or your hand as a guide for appropriate portion sizes. Start with smaller portions and add more if you're still feeling hungry after a reasonable amount of time.
- **Read Food Labels:** Pay attention to serving sizes on food labels. This helps you stay mindful of calorie and nutrient intake.

Sample Meal Plans for Different Dietary Needs:

This section provides a springboard for creating your personalized meal plan. We offer sample plans for different dietary needs, keeping in mind the principles of a balanced plate and anti-inflammatory ingredients:

- **Breakfast:** Scrambled eggs with spinach and smoked salmon, whole-wheat toast with avocado
- **Lunch:** Chopped salad with grilled chicken, quinoa, and a balsamic vinaigrette
- **Dinner:** Baked salmon with roasted vegetables, brown rice
- **Snacks:** Greek yogurt with berries and chia seeds, handful of almonds

Sample Meal Plan (Vegetarian):

- **Breakfast:** Oatmeal with berries and walnuts
- **Lunch:** Lentil soup with whole-wheat bread
- **Dinner:** Black bean burgers on whole-wheat buns with sweet potato fries
- **Snacks:** Edamame with a sprinkle of sea salt, apple slices with almond butter

Sample Meal Plan (Gluten-Free):

- **Breakfast:** Frittata with vegetables and cheese (choose gluten-free cheese if needed), gluten-free toast with nut butter
- **Lunch:** Tuna salad with chopped vegetables on romaine lettuce wraps

- **Dinner:** Chicken stir-fry with brown rice noodles and vegetables
- **Snacks:** Fruit salad with coconut yogurt, sliced vegetables with hummus

PART 2 DELICIOUS RECIPES FOR RELIEF

CHAPTER 4

STARTING YOUR DAY RIGHT - FUELING YOUR BODY FOR AN ACTIVE MORNING WITH PMR

Breakfast is often called the most important meal of the day, and for those managing Polymyalgia Rheumatica (PMR), it holds even greater significance. A well-balanced and anti-inflammatory breakfast sets the tone for the day, providing sustained energy, promoting satiety, and potentially reducing stiffness and pain associated with PMR. Let's explore some delicious and nutritious breakfast options to kickstart your mornings:

Omega-3 Powerhouse - Scrambled Eggs with Smoked Salmon and Spinach

This recipe combines the goodness of protein-rich eggs with omega-3 fatty acids from smoked salmon and the anti-inflammatory power of spinach.

Ingredients:

- 2 large eggs
- 1 tablespoon unsweetened almond milk (or milk of your choice)
- 1/4 cup chopped fresh spinach
- 2 ounces smoked salmon, flaked
- 1 tablespoon olive oil
- Salt and freshly ground black pepper to taste
- Optional additions: Chopped chives, crumbled feta cheese (if tolerated)

Instructions:

1. In a bowl, whisk together eggs and almond milk (or milk of your choice) until well combined. Season with a pinch of salt and pepper.
2. Heat olive oil in a non-stick pan over medium heat. Add the spinach and cook until wilted, about 1 minute.
3. Pour the egg mixture into the pan and scramble with a spatula until cooked through to your desired consistency.
4. Remove from heat and fold in the smoked salmon.
5. Serve immediately on a plate. Garnish with chopped chives and crumbled feta cheese (optional).

Nutritional Facts (per serving):

- Calories: 300
- Protein: 18g
- Fat: 18g (including 5g omega-3 fatty acids)
- Carbohydrates: 4g
- Fiber: 1g

Tips:

- For a creamier texture, use whole eggs instead of just egg whites.
- Add a squeeze of lemon juice to the scrambled eggs for a touch of brightness.
- If you don't have fresh spinach, you can use frozen spinach, thawed and squeezed dry.

Berrylicious Smoothie - Packed with Antioxidants and Chia Seeds for Fiber

This refreshing smoothie is a quick and convenient way to start your day with a burst of anti-inflammatory antioxidants from berries and the added benefit of fiber-rich chia seeds.

Ingredients:

- 1 cup frozen mixed berries (blueberries, raspberries, strawberries)
- 1 cup unsweetened almond milk (or milk of your choice)
- 1/2 banana, frozen
- 1 tablespoon chia seeds
- 1 scoop protein powder (optional, choose unsweetened and unflavored if following a specific dietary restriction)
- 1/4 cup plain Greek yogurt (optional)
- Pinch of ground cinnamon

Instructions:

1. Combine all ingredients in a blender and blend until smooth and creamy.
2. Add a splash of water or more almond milk if the smoothie is too thick.
3. Pour into a glass and enjoy!

Nutritional Facts (per serving, without protein powder or Greek yogurt):

- Calories: 180
- Protein: 2g
- Fat: 4g
- Carbohydrates: 30g

- Fiber: 5g

Tips:

- Feel free to experiment with different types of frozen fruits like mango or pineapple.
- Add a handful of spinach for an extra boost of nutrients.
- If you prefer a thicker smoothie, use less almond milk or add more frozen banana.

Additional Recipe Ideas:

1. **Oatmeal with Fruit and Nuts:** A classic breakfast option packed with fiber and healthy fats. Choose steel-cut oats for a more sustained release of energy. Top with berries, sliced banana, and a sprinkle of almonds or walnuts.
2. **Chia Pudding with Berries:** This overnight oats alternative is perfect for meal prepping. Combine chia seeds, almond milk, and a touch of honey in a jar, refrigerate overnight, and top with fresh berries in the morning.

CHAPTER 5

LIGHT AND NOURISHING LUNCHES - POWERING THROUGH YOUR AFTERNOON WITH PMR

Lunchtime is a crucial opportunity to refuel your body and mind after a busy morning. For those managing Polymyalgia Rheumatica (PMR), choosing a light yet nourishing lunch can help maintain energy levels, reduce stiffness, and support overall well-being. This chapter explores delicious and anti-inflammatory lunch options that are easy to prepare and perfect for packing or enjoying at home.

Mediterranean Feast - Salmon Salad with Chopped Vegetables and Olive Oil Dressing

This vibrant salad combines protein-rich salmon with a variety of colorful vegetables, all drizzled with a heart-healthy olive oil dressing, for a satisfying and anti-inflammatory lunch.

Ingredients:

- 4 ounces cooked salmon, flaked (grilled, baked, poached, or canned)
- 2 cups mixed greens (spinach, arugula, romaine)
- 1/2 cup chopped cherry tomatoes
- 1/2 cucumber, sliced
- 1/4 cup crumbled feta cheese (optional, if tolerated)
- 1/4 cup Kalamata olives, pitted and halved

For the Dressing:

- 2 tablespoons extra virgin olive oil
- 1 tablespoon lemon juice
- 1 teaspoon Dijon mustard
- 1/2 teaspoon dried oregano
- Salt and freshly ground black pepper to taste

Instructions:

1. In a large bowl, combine mixed greens, cherry tomatoes, cucumber, feta cheese (if using), and Kalamata olives.
2. Top with flaked salmon.
3. In a small bowl, whisk together olive oil, lemon juice, Dijon mustard, oregano, salt, and pepper.

4. Drizzle the dressing over the salad and toss to coat.
5. Serve immediately.

Nutritional Facts (per serving, without feta cheese):

- Calories: 400
- Protein: 30g
- Fat: 18g (including healthy fats from olive oil)
- Carbohydrates: 15g
- Fiber: 4g

Tips:

- Leftover grilled, baked, poached, or even canned salmon can be used for this recipe.
- Feel free to add other chopped vegetables like bell peppers, red onion, or chopped fennel for additional flavor and texture.
- If you don't have Dijon mustard, you can substitute it with another type of mustard or a drizzle of balsamic vinegar.

Leafy Green Goodness - Spinach Salad with Walnuts, Berries, and Goat Cheese (modify cheese if needed)

This salad is a powerhouse of anti-inflammatory ingredients. Spinach provides essential vitamins and minerals, walnuts offer healthy fats, and berries add a touch of sweetness and antioxidants.

Ingredients:

- 4 cups baby spinach
- 1/2 cup walnuts, toasted and chopped
- 1/2 cup blueberries or raspberries
- 1/4 cup crumbled goat cheese (modify cheese if needed due to dietary restrictions)
- **For the Dressing:**
- 2 tablespoons olive oil
- 1 tablespoon balsamic vinegar
- 1 teaspoon honey
- 1/2 teaspoon Dijon mustard
- Salt and freshly ground black pepper to taste

Instructions:

1. In a large bowl, combine spinach, walnuts, and berries.

2. Crumble goat cheese over the salad.
3. In a small bowl, whisk together olive oil, balsamic vinegar, honey, Dijon mustard, salt, and pepper.
4. Drizzle the dressing over the salad and toss to coat.
5. Serve immediately.

Nutritional Facts (per serving):

- Calories: 350
- Protein: 8g
- Fat: 20g (including healthy fats from walnuts)
- Carbohydrates: 25g
- Fiber: 5g

Tips:

- You can substitute the goat cheese with crumbled feta cheese (if tolerated) or another type of cheese that fits your dietary needs.
- Add a grilled chicken breast or a scoop of cooked lentils for additional protein.
- Drizzle the salad with a sprinkle of balsamic glaze for a touch of sweetness and complexity.

Anti-Inflammatory Wrap - Turkey and Veggie Wrap with Whole-Wheat Tortilla

This wrap is a portable and protein-packed lunch option, perfect for busy days. The combination of whole-wheat tortillas, lean turkey, and a variety of vegetables provides sustained energy and essential nutrients.

Ingredients:

- 1 whole-wheat tortilla
- 3 ounces sliced turkey breast
- 1/2 cup chopped romaine lettuce
- 1/4 cup chopped cucumber
- 1/4 cup shredded carrots
- 1/4 cup hummus (choose a variety without added sugars)
- 1 tablespoon chopped red onion (optional)
- Salt and freshly ground black pepper to taste

Instructions:

1. Spread hummus evenly over the whole-wheat tortilla.
2. Layer romaine lettuce, cucumber, shredded carrots, red onion (if using), and sliced turkey breast.
3. Season with salt and pepper to taste.
4. Roll up the tortilla tightly, starting from one end.

5. Cut the wrap in half for easier handling (optional).
6. Serve immediately.

Nutritional Facts (per serving):

- Calories: 350
- Protein: 25g
- Fat: 10g (including healthy fats from hummus)
- Carbohydrates: 30g
- Fiber: 5g

Tips:

- Experiment with different fillings like grilled chicken breast, shredded salmon, or tofu scramble for a vegetarian option.
- Add a dollop of plain Greek yogurt for an extra protein boost.
- Include a side of sliced bell peppers or baby carrots for additional vegetable intake.

Additional Recipe Ideas:

Lentil Soup: This hearty soup is a great source of plant-based protein and fiber. It's perfect for a cold winter day and can be easily made in a slow cooker. Here's a simple recipe:

Ingredients:

- 1 cup brown lentils, rinsed; 4 cups vegetable broth;
- 1 onion, chopped; 2 carrots, chopped; 2 celery stalks, chopped; 2 cloves garlic, minced; 1 teaspoon dried thyme;
- 1 teaspoon ground cumin; Salt and freshly ground black pepper to taste.

Instructions:

- Saute onion, carrots, and celery in a large pot with a drizzle of olive oil until softened.
- Add garlic, thyme, and cumin, cook for an additional minute. Stir in lentils, vegetable broth, and bring to a boil.
- Reduce heat, simmer for 30-40 minutes or until lentils are tender. Season with salt and pepper to taste.

- ✓ **Chickpea Salad Sandwich on Whole-Wheat Bread:** This vegetarian option is packed with protein and fiber. Mash cooked chickpeas with chopped celery, red onion, a light mayonnaise dressing, and your favorite herbs and spices. Spread on whole-wheat bread and enjoy!

CHAPTER 6

FLAVORFUL AND SATISFYING DINNERS - NOURISHING YOUR BODY FOR A RESTFUL NIGHT WITH PMR

As the day comes to a close, a nourishing and anti-inflammatory dinner sets the stage for a restful night's sleep and supports your overall well-being with PMR. This chapter dives into delicious and satisfying dinner recipes that are easy to prepare and perfect for weeknights or special occasions.

One-Pan Wonder - Roasted Salmon with Vegetables and Herbs

This recipe is a one-pan marvel, minimizing cleanup and maximizing flavor. Salmon, rich in omega-3 fatty acids, is roasted with colorful vegetables, infused with the aroma of fresh herbs.

Ingredients:

- 2 salmon fillets (each about 6 ounces)
- 1 tablespoon olive oil
- 1/2 teaspoon dried oregano
- 1/4 teaspoon garlic powder
- Salt and freshly ground black pepper to taste
- 1 medium zucchini, sliced
- 1 red bell pepper, sliced
- 1 yellow bell pepper, sliced
- 1/2 red onion, sliced
- 1 cup cherry tomatoes
- 1/4 cup chopped fresh parsley (for garnish)

Instructions:

1. Preheat oven to 400°F (200°C). Line a baking sheet with parchment paper.
2. In a small bowl, combine olive oil, oregano, garlic powder, salt, and pepper.
3. Place salmon fillets on the prepared baking sheet. Brush the salmon with the olive oil mixture.
4. Scatter zucchini slices, bell pepper slices, red onion slices, and cherry tomatoes around the salmon.

5. Roast for 20-25 minutes, or until the salmon is cooked through and flakes easily with a fork, and the vegetables are tender-crisp.
6. Garnish with fresh parsley before serving.

Nutritional Facts (per serving):

- Calories: 450
- Protein: 35g
- Fat: 20g (including healthy fats from salmon and olive oil)
- Carbohydrates: 25g
- Fiber: 4g

Tips:

- Substitute other types of fish like cod or halibut for salmon.
- Feel free to add other vegetables like broccoli florets or asparagus spears.
- For a more robust flavor profile, marinate the salmon in the olive oil mixture for 15 minutes before baking.
- Leftovers can be stored in an airtight container in the refrigerator for up to 3 days.

Veggie Power Bowl - Quinoa Bowl with Roasted Vegetables and Tahini Dressing

This vibrant bowl is packed with protein, fiber, and a variety of vitamins and minerals from the roasted vegetables. The tahini dressing adds a creamy and flavorful touch.

Ingredients:

- 1 cup quinoa, rinsed
- 1.5 cups vegetable broth
- 1 tablespoon olive oil
- 1/2 teaspoon dried thyme
- Salt and freshly ground black pepper to taste
- 1 cup broccoli florets
- 1 red bell pepper, sliced
- 1 yellow bell pepper, sliced
- 1/2 red onion, sliced
- 1 tablespoon olive oil (for roasting vegetables)

For the Tahini Dressing:

- 2 tablespoons tahini
- 2 tablespoons lemon juice
- 1 tablespoon water
- 1 clove garlic, minced

- 1/4 cup chopped fresh parsley
- Salt and freshly ground black pepper to taste

Instructions:

1. Preheat oven to 400°F (200°C). Line a baking sheet with parchment paper.
2. In a medium saucepan, combine quinoa, vegetable broth, 1 tablespoon olive oil, thyme, salt, and pepper. Bring to a boil, then reduce heat, cover, and simmer for 15 minutes, or until quinoa is cooked and fluffy.
3. Toss broccoli florets, bell pepper slices, and red onion slices with 1 tablespoon olive oil. Spread the vegetables on the prepared baking sheet and roast for 20-25 minutes, or until tender-crisp.
4. While the vegetables are roasting, prepare the tahini dressing. In a small bowl, whisk together tahini, lemon juice, water, garlic, parsley, salt, and pepper.
5. To assemble the bowls, divide cooked quinoa among serving plates. Top with roasted vegetables and drizzle with tahini dressing.

Nutritional Facts (per serving):

- Calories: 400

- Protein: 12g
- Fat: 15g (including healthy fats from tahini)
- Carbohydrates: 50g
- Fiber: 8g

Tips:

- Experiment with different roasted vegetables like Brussels sprouts, sweet potato cubes, or butternut squash.

Anti-Inflammatory Pasta Delight - Whole-Wheat Pasta with Shrimp and Spinach Pesto

This recipe combines the goodness of whole-wheat pasta with protein-rich shrimp and a vibrant spinach pesto, creating a delicious and anti-inflammatory dinner option.

Ingredients:

- 8 ounces whole-wheat pasta
- 1 tablespoon olive oil
- 1 shallot, minced
- 2 cloves garlic, minced
- 4 ounces raw shrimp, peeled and deveined
- 4 cups baby spinach

- 1/2 cup pine nuts (toasted, optional)
- 1/4 cup grated Parmesan cheese (or dairy-free alternative if needed)
- 1/4 cup olive oil
- Salt and freshly ground black pepper to taste

Instructions:

1. Cook whole-wheat pasta according to package instructions. Drain and set aside.
2. While the pasta is cooking, heat olive oil in a large skillet over medium heat. Add shallot and garlic, cook for 2-3 minutes, or until softened.
3. Add shrimp to the pan and cook for 3-4 minutes, or until pink and opaque. Remove shrimp from the pan and set aside.
4. In a food processor, combine spinach, pine nuts (if using), Parmesan cheese, olive oil, salt, and pepper. Pulse until a coarse pesto forms.
5. In a large bowl, toss cooked pasta with the spinach pesto and cooked shrimp.
6. Serve immediately and enjoy!

Nutritional Facts (per serving):

- Calories: 500
- Protein: 30g
- Fat: 20g (including healthy fats from olive oil and pine nuts)
- Carbohydrates: 50g
- Fiber: 4g

Tips:

- If you don't have pine nuts, you can substitute them with another type of nut or seed like walnuts or sunflower seeds.
- For a vegetarian option, omit the shrimp and add a cup of cooked chickpeas or lentils to the pasta.
- Leftovers can be stored in an airtight container in the refrigerator for up to 3 days.

Additional Recipe Ideas:

- ✓ **Chicken Stir-Fry with Vegetables:** A quick and customizable option. Marinate chicken strips in a mixture of soy sauce, ginger, garlic, and a touch of honey. Stir-fry with colorful vegetables like broccoli, bell peppers, and snow peas. Serve over brown rice or quinoa.
- ✓ **Vegetarian Chili:** A hearty and comforting dish perfect for a cold winter night. Combine kidney beans, black beans,

corn, diced tomatoes, and your favorite chili spices in a slow cooker. Let it simmer for a few hours and enjoy with a side of chopped avocado and a dollop of plain Greek yogurt.

CHAPTER 7

SMART SNACKING FOR SUSTAINED ENERGY - POWERING THROUGH YOUR DAY WITH PMR

Healthy snacking is a crucial part of managing Polymyalgia Rheumatica (PMR). Choosing the right snacks can help maintain energy levels throughout the day, reduce inflammation, and support overall well-being. This chapter explores delicious and convenient snack options that are packed with essential nutrients and can be enjoyed between meals or on the go.

Trail Mix Powerhouse - Homemade Trail Mix with Nuts, Seeds, and Dried Fruit (modify based on tolerated ingredients)
This customizable trail mix provides a delightful combination of protein, healthy fats, fiber, and antioxidants. It's a perfect grab-and-go snack that keeps you feeling energized and satisfied.

Ingredients:

- 1/2 cup raw almonds

- 1/4 cup raw cashews
- 1/4 cup pumpkin seeds
- 1/4 cup dried cranberries (or raisins if tolerated)
- 1/4 cup dried cherries (or chopped dried apricots if tolerated)
- 1/4 cup unsweetened shredded coconut (optional)

Instructions:

1. In a medium bowl, combine all ingredients.
2. Mix well and store in an airtight container at room temperature.

Nutritional Facts (per 1/2 cup serving):

- Calories: 300
- Protein: 6g
- Fat: 15g (including healthy fats from nuts and seeds)
- Carbohydrates: 25g
- Fiber: 4g

Tips:

- Feel free to adjust the ingredients based on your preferences and dietary needs.

- You can include other nuts like walnuts or pecans, seeds like sunflower seeds or flaxseeds, and dried fruits like dried figs or goji berries (if tolerated).
- To avoid added sugars, choose unsweetened dried fruits or make your own by dehydrating fresh fruits at home.
- Portion control is key. Store the trail mix in individual containers to avoid overindulging.

Energy Bites - Antioxidant-Rich Energy Bites with Dates, Nuts, and Seeds

These no-bake energy bites are packed with flavor and nutrition. Dates provide natural sweetness, while nuts and seeds offer protein, healthy fats, and antioxidants.

Ingredients:

- 1 cup pitted medjool dates
- 1/2 cup rolled oats
- 1/4 cup chopped walnuts
- 1/4 cup chopped almonds
- 1/4 cup chia seeds
- 2 tablespoons unsweetened shredded coconut (optional)
- 1 teaspoon vanilla extract

Instructions:

1. In a food processor, pulse together dates, rolled oats, walnuts, almonds, chia seeds, and shredded coconut (if using) until a sticky mixture forms.
2. Stir in vanilla extract and pulse a few more times to combine.
3. Roll the mixture into tablespoon-sized balls.
4. Store energy bites in an airtight container in the refrigerator for up to a week.

Nutritional Facts (per 1 energy bite):

- Calories: 150
- Protein: 3g
- Fat: 7g (including healthy fats from nuts and seeds)
- Carbohydrates: 20g
- Fiber: 2g

Tips:

- Experiment with different nut and seed combinations to create your own flavor variations.
- For a more decadent touch, roll the energy bites in unsweetened cocoa powder or shredded coconut.

- If the mixture feels too dry, add a tablespoon of almond butter or coconut oil.

Yogurt Delight - Greek Yogurt with Berries and Chia Seeds

This simple yet satisfying snack combines protein-rich Greek yogurt with the sweetness and antioxidants of berries and the added benefits of chia seeds.

Ingredients:

- 1 cup plain Greek yogurt (2% or higher fat content)
- 1/2 cup fresh berries (blueberries, raspberries, strawberries, or a mix)
- 2 tablespoons chia seeds

Instructions:

1. In a bowl, combine Greek yogurt, berries, and chia seeds.
2. Stir gently and enjoy!

Nutritional Facts (per serving):

- Calories: 200

- Protein: 20g
- Fat: 5g (including healthy fats from yogurt)
- Carbohydrates: 20g
- Fiber: 4g (including fiber from chia seeds)

Tips:

- Use flavored Greek yogurt if plain yogurt is too tart for your taste. However, be mindful of added sugars and choose options with minimal sugar content.
- For added texture, top your yogurt with a sprinkle of chopped nuts or granola (choose a low-sugar option).
- Frozen berries can be used instead of fresh ones. Let them thaw slightly before adding them to
- the yogurt for a chilled and refreshing snack.

Additional Recipe Ideas:

- ✓ **Hard-Boiled Eggs:** A classic and convenient source of protein. Hard-boiled eggs are easy to prepare in advance and can be enjoyed on their own or sliced and added to salads or sandwiches.
- ✓ **Sliced Vegetables with Hummus:** This colorful and healthy snack is packed with fiber and healthy fats. Choose a variety of colorful vegetables like carrots, bell peppers,

cucumber slices, and cherry tomatoes. Pair them with a portion of hummus for a satisfying and dippable snack.

maintain steady energy levels and support your overall well-being with PMR.

PART 3: LIVING WELL WITH POLYMYALGIA RHEUMATICA

CHAPTER 8

ADDITIONAL TIPS FOR MANAGING POLYMYALGIA RHEUMATICA - OPTIMIZING YOUR WELL-BEING BEYOND DIET

While a healthy diet plays a crucial role in managing Polymyalgia Rheumatica (PMR), a holistic approach is essential for optimal well-being. This chapter explores additional lifestyle practices that can significantly improve your quality of life and empower you to manage PMR effectively.

1. Importance of Exercise and Movement:

Regular exercise, even in modified forms, is crucial for managing PMR symptoms. Gentle movement helps maintain muscle strength, flexibility, and range of motion, which can improve stiffness and reduce pain. Here are some tips for incorporating exercise into your PMR routine:

- ✓ **Start Low and Slow:** Begin with low-impact exercises like walking, swimming, or water aerobics. Gradually increase the intensity and duration of your workouts as your tolerance improves.
- ✓ **Listen to Your Body:** Pay attention to your pain levels and adjust your exercise routine accordingly. Don't push yourself through pain, as this can worsen symptoms.
- ✓ **Warm-Up and Cool-Down:** Always perform gentle stretches before and after exercise to loosen muscles and reduce the risk of injury.
- ✓ **Consider Physical Therapy:** A physical therapist can create a personalized exercise program tailored to your specific needs and limitations. They can also teach you proper techniques and stretches to maximize benefits and minimize pain.

2. Prioritizing Sleep and Relaxation Techniques:

Adequate sleep is vital for overall health and plays a significant role in managing PMR symptoms. During sleep, your body repairs tissues and regulates inflammation. Here are some tips for promoting restful sleep:

- ✓ **Establish a Regular Sleep Schedule:** Go to bed and wake up at consistent times each day, even on weekends. This helps regulate your body's natural sleep-wake cycle.
- ✓ **Create a Relaxing Bedtime Routine:** Wind down before bed with calming activities like reading, taking a warm bath, or practicing relaxation techniques like deep breathing or meditation.
- ✓ **Optimize Your Sleep Environment:** Make sure your bedroom is dark, quiet, and cool. Invest in a comfortable mattress and pillows to promote better sleep quality.
- ✓ **Manage Stress:** Chronic stress can disrupt sleep patterns and worsen PMR symptoms. Practice relaxation techniques like yoga, meditation, or deep breathing to manage stress and promote better sleep.

3. Importance of Hydration:

Staying hydrated is vital for overall health and can help manage PMR symptoms. Dehydration can lead to stiffness and fatigue, making PMR symptoms worse. Here are some tips for staying hydrated:

- ✓ **Drink Plenty of Water Throughout the Day:** Aim for eight glasses of water per day as a baseline, but adjust based on your individual needs and activity level.

- ✓ **Choose Water-Rich Beverages:** Include herbal tea, unsweetened green tea, or diluted fruit juices in your daily intake.
- ✓ **Eat Water-Rich Foods:** Incorporate fruits and vegetables like watermelon, celery, cucumber, and leafy greens into your diet, as they contribute to your daily fluid intake.
- ✓ **Monitor Your Urine Color:** Aim for pale yellow urine, indicating adequate hydration. Darker urine suggests dehydration.

4. The Mind-Body Connection: Stress Management and Emotional Wellbeing:

Chronic stress can exacerbate PMR symptoms and negatively impact your overall well-being. Learning to manage stress effectively is essential for managing PMR. Here are some tips for promoting emotional well-being:

- ✓ **Practice Relaxation Techniques:** Regularly incorporate stress-relieving practices like yoga, meditation, or deep breathing exercises into your routine.
- ✓ **Connect with Others:** Social support is crucial. Talk to supportive friends, family members, or a therapist about your challenges and emotions.

- ✓ **Focus on Gratitude:** Practicing gratitude by focusing on the positive aspects of your life can improve your mood and overall well-being.
- ✓ **Mindfulness Techniques:** Mindfulness exercises can help you stay present in the moment and reduce anxiety. Consider guided meditations or mindfulness walks.
- ✓ **Seek Professional Help:** If stress or anxiety is overwhelming, don't hesitate to seek professional help from a therapist or counselor.
- ✓ **Remember:** Managing PMR is a journey, not a destination. By incorporating these additional tips into your lifestyle, alongside a healthy diet, you can effectively manage your symptoms, improve your quality of life, and empower yourself to take control of your health and well-being.

CHAPTER 9

BUILDING A SUPPORT SYSTEM - A NETWORK FOR STRENGTH AND SHARED EXPERIENCES WITH PMR

Navigating life with PMR can be challenging. Building a strong support system is crucial for emotional well-being and effective disease management. This chapter explores the importance of communication with your healthcare team and the benefits of connecting with others who understand the unique challenges of PMR.

1. Communicating with Your Doctor and Healthcare Team:
Open and honest communication with your doctor and healthcare team is the cornerstone of effective PMR management. Here are some tips for maximizing your doctor visits:

- ✓ **Prepare a List of Questions and Concerns:** Write down your questions and concerns beforehand, so you don't forget anything during your appointment. This includes specific questions about PMR symptoms, medication side effects, and treatment options.

✓ **Track Your Symptoms:** Keep a journal to track your symptoms, including pain levels, stiffness duration, and any changes you experience. Bringing this record to your doctor's appointments can provide valuable insights.

✓ **Be an Active Participant:** Don't hesitate to ask for clarification or express your concerns. The more information you share, the better equipped your doctor is to manage your condition effectively.

✓ **Build a Collaborative Relationship:** View your doctor as a partner in your healthcare journey. Work together to develop a treatment plan that fits your specific needs and preferences.

✓ **Advocate for Yourself:** Don't be afraid to ask questions and express your concerns. You are your biggest health advocate.

✓ **Build Trust with Your Care Team:** A strong relationship with your doctor and healthcare team fosters trust and allows you to feel comfortable expressing your needs and concerns openly.

2. **The Power of Support Groups and Online Communities:**

Connecting with others who understand the challenges of PMR can be a source of strength, encouragement, and valuable information.

- ✓ **Support Groups:** Joining a PMR support group can connect you with individuals facing similar experiences. These groups offer a safe space to share your experiences, seek and offer advice, and learn from each other's coping mechanisms.
- ✓ Consider both in-person and online support groups to find one that best fits your needs and preferences.
- ✓ Inquire with your doctor or local hospitals about PMR support groups in your area. Support group directories and online resources can also be helpful in finding a group.
- ✓ **Online Communities:** Online forums and social media groups dedicated to PMR can provide a wealth of information, support, and a sense of community.
- ✓ Choose reputable online communities with credible information and active participation.
- ✓ Be mindful of the information you share online and prioritize reliable sources for medical advice.

Additional Tips:

Support groups and online communities can be helpful for both patients and caregivers.

Consider attending support group meetings with a loved one or caregiver for additional support.

If you experience challenges finding a support group in your area, online resources and virtual support groups can be valuable alternatives.

By establishing a strong support network and fostering open communication with your healthcare team, you can create a foundation for successful PMR management and a more fulfilling journey towards optimal well-being.

CHAPTER 10

A LOOK TO THE FUTURE: MAINTAINING A POSITIVE OUTLOOK WITH PMR

Living with Polymyalgia Rheumatica (PMR) can present challenges, but it doesn't have to define your future. By adopting a positive outlook and focusing on self-care strategies, you can lead a fulfilling and active life. This chapter explores strategies for cultivating optimism, managing stress, and embracing a proactive approach to your health.

1. The Power of Positive Thinking:

A positive outlook is a powerful tool for managing PMR. Here are some ways to cultivate optimism:

- ✓ **Focus on Gratitude:** Shift your focus towards the things you are grateful for, big or small. Taking time to appreciate the positive aspects of your life can significantly improve your mood and overall well-being.

- ✓ **Practice Positive Self-Talk:** Challenge negative thoughts and replace them with encouraging affirmations. Focus on your strengths and capabilities rather than dwelling on limitations.
- ✓ **Visualize Success:** Imagine yourself achieving your health goals and living a fulfilling life with PMR. Positive visualization can be a powerful tool for boosting motivation and resilience.
- ✓ **Celebrate Small Victories:** Acknowledge and celebrate your progress, no matter how small. Every step forward is a victory in managing your condition.
- ✓ **Focus on What You Can Control:** While you can't control the presence of PMR, you can control your response to it. Focus your energy on the aspects of your health and life that you can influence.

2. Effective Stress Management:

Chronic stress can exacerbate PMR symptoms and negatively impact your overall well-being. Here are some stress-management techniques you can incorporate into your daily routine:

- ✓ **Relaxation Techniques:** Regularly practice relaxation techniques like deep breathing exercises, meditation, or progressive muscle relaxation. These practices can help calm your mind and body, reducing stress and promoting feelings of peace.

- ✓ **Mindfulness Practices:** Mindfulness exercises encourage you to stay present in the moment and let go of worries about the future or regrets about the past. Consider guided meditations or mindfulness walks to cultivate present-moment awareness.
- ✓ **Physical Activity:** Regular exercise, even in modified forms, is a powerful stress reliever. Walking, swimming, yoga, and gentle stretching can all help manage stress and improve your mood.
- ✓ **Engage in Activities You Enjoy:** Make time for activities you find pleasurable, whether it's reading, spending time in nature, listening to music, or pursuing hobbies. Engaging in enjoyable activities can significantly reduce stress and improve your overall well-being.
- ✓ **Seek Support:** Don't hesitate to reach out to friends, family members, or a therapist for support when you're feeling overwhelmed. Talking about your challenges can be a powerful stress reliever.

3. Embracing a Proactive Approach:

Taking a proactive approach to your health empowers you to manage PMR effectively. Here are some ways to stay engaged in your healthcare journey:

- ✓ **Stay Informed:** Educate yourself about PMR, treatment options, and potential side effects. Reliable sources include patient education websites, reputable medical journals, and information provided by your doctor.
- ✓ **Track Your Symptoms:** Monitoring your symptoms can help you identify patterns and triggers. Keeping a symptom journal can be a valuable tool in communicating with your doctor and making informed decisions about your treatment plan.
- ✓ **Maintain Regular Doctor Visits:** Don't skip your doctor appointments. Regular checkups are essential for monitoring your condition, adjusting treatment plans as needed, and addressing any concerns you may have.
- ✓ **Participate in Your Treatment Plan:** Actively participate in discussions about your treatment plan with your doctor. Ask questions, express your concerns, and work collaboratively to find a treatment approach that works best for you.

✓ **Explore Complementary Therapies:** Consider incorporating complementary therapies like acupuncture, massage therapy, or tai chi into your routine, alongside conventional treatment plans. These practices can potentially improve pain management and promote overall well-being. However, discuss any complementary therapies with your doctor first to ensure they are safe and appropriate for you.

Remember:

Maintaining a positive outlook is a journey, not a destination. There will be good days and bad days, but focusing on self-care and staying positive can significantly improve your overall well-being.

You are not alone. Many people live fulfilling lives with PMR. By adopting a proactive approach and fostering a strong support network, you can effectively manage your condition and create a life filled with purpose and joy.

BONUS CHAPTER

BONUS RECIPES FOR POLYMYALGIA RHEUMATIC DIET

Flavorful and Satisfying Dinners - Nourishing Your Body for a Restful Night with PMR

As the day comes to a close, a nourishing and anti-inflammatory dinner sets the stage for a restful night's sleep and supports your overall well-being with PMR. This chapter dives into delicious and satisfying dinner recipes that are easy to prepare and perfect for weeknights or special occasions.

One-Pan Wonder - Roasted Salmon with Spinach and Tomatoes

Ingredients:

- 2 salmon fillets (each about 6 ounces)
- 1 tablespoon olive oil
- 1/2 teaspoon dried oregano
- 1/4 teaspoon garlic powder
- Salt and freshly ground black pepper to taste
- 1 cup cherry tomatoes
- 4 cups baby spinach

Instructions:

1. Preheat oven to 400°F (200°C). Line a baking sheet with parchment paper.
2. In a small bowl, combine olive oil, oregano, garlic powder, salt, and pepper.
3. Place salmon fillets on the prepared baking sheet. Brush the salmon with the olive oil mixture.
4. Scatter cherry tomatoes around the salmon.
5. Roast for 15-20 minutes, or until the salmon is cooked through and flakes easily with a fork, and the tomatoes are blistered.
6. In the last 2 minutes of cooking, add the baby spinach to the baking sheet and let it wilt slightly.
7. Serve immediately and enjoy!

Nutritional Facts (per serving):

- Calories: 400
- Protein: 35g
- Fat: 20g (including healthy fats from salmon and olive oil)
- Carbohydrates: 20g
- Fiber: 4g

Tips

- Substitute other types of fish like cod or halibut for salmon.
- Feel free to add other vegetables like sliced bell peppers or zucchini.
- For extra flavor, marinate the salmon in the olive oil mixture for 15 minutes before baking.
- Leftovers can be stored in an airtight container in the refrigerator for up to 3 days.

Protein Power Bowl - Quinoa with Roasted Vegetables and Almonds

Ingredients:

- 1 cup quinoa, rinsed
- 1.5 cups vegetable broth
- 1 tablespoon olive oil
- 1/2 teaspoon dried thyme
- Salt and freshly ground black pepper to taste
- 1 cup broccoli florets
- 1 red bell pepper, sliced
- 1/2 red onion, sliced
- 1/4 cup sliced almonds

Instructions:

1. Preheat oven to 400°F (200°C). Line a baking sheet with parchment paper.
2. In a medium saucepan, combine quinoa, vegetable broth, 1 tablespoon olive oil, thyme, salt, and pepper. Bring to a boil, then reduce heat, cover, and simmer for 15 minutes, or until quinoa is cooked and fluffy.
3. Toss broccoli florets, bell pepper slices, and red onion slices with a drizzle of olive oil. Spread the vegetables on the prepared baking sheet and roast for 20-25 minutes, or until tender-crisp.
4. While the vegetables are roasting, toast the almonds in a dry skillet over medium heat until fragrant, watching closely to avoid burning.
5. To assemble the bowls, divide cooked quinoa among serving plates. Top with roasted vegetables and toasted almonds.

Nutritional Facts (per serving):

- Calories: 450
- Protein: 15g
- Fat: 18g (including healthy fats from almonds and olive oil)
- Carbohydrates: 55g
- Fiber: 8g

Tips:

- Experiment with different roasted vegetables like Brussels sprouts, sweet potato cubes, or butternut squash.
- For added protein, sprinkle cooked chickpeas or lentils on top of the quinoa.
- Use chopped walnuts or pecans instead of almonds.
- Leftovers can be stored in an airtight container in the refrigerator for up to 3 days.

Sheet Pan Frittata with Spinach and Cherry Tomatoes

Ingredients:

- 8 eggs
- 1/4 cup milk (unsweetened almond milk or low-fat
- 1/4 cup chopped fresh spinach
- 1/2 cup cherry tomatoes, halved
- 1/4 cup crumbled feta cheese (optional)
- 1/4 cup chopped fresh parsley
- 1/4 teaspoon dried oregano
- Salt and freshly ground black pepper to taste
- 1 tablespoon olive oil

Instructions:

1. Preheat oven to 400°F (200°C). Line a baking sheet with parchment paper.
2. In a large bowl, whisk together eggs, milk, spinach, cherry tomatoes (reserve a few for garnish), feta cheese (if using), parsley, oregano, salt, and pepper.
3. Pour the egg mixture onto the prepared baking sheet. Drizzle with olive oil.
4. Scatter the reserved cherry tomatoes on top.
5. Bake for 20-25 minutes, or until the eggs are set and the center is no longer runny.
6. Let cool slightly before slicing and serving.

Nutritional Facts (per serving, without feta cheese):

- Calories: 250
- Protein: 18g
- Fat: 12g (including healthy fats from olive oil)
- Carbohydrates: 10g
- Fiber: 2g

Tips:

- For a vegetarian option, omit the feta cheese.
- Add other chopped vegetables like bell peppers, onions, or mushrooms to the egg mixture.

- Leftovers can be stored in an airtight container in the refrigerator for up to 3 days and enjoyed for breakfast or lunch.

Spiced Salmon with Berry Salsa

Ingredients:

- 2 salmon fillets (each about 6 ounces)
- 1 tablespoon olive oil
- 1/2 teaspoon paprika
- 1/4 teaspoon chili powder
- 1/4 teaspoon garlic powder
- Salt and freshly ground black pepper to taste
- 1 cup mixed berries (such as strawberries, blueberries, raspberries)
- 1/4 cup chopped red onion
- 1 tablespoon lime juice
- 1/4 cup chopped fresh cilantro
- Pinch of red pepper flakes (optional)

Instructions

1. Preheat oven to 400°F (200°C). Line a baking sheet with parchment paper.

2. In a small bowl, combine olive oil, paprika, chili powder, garlic powder, salt, and pepper.
3. Rub the spice mixture onto both sides of the salmon fillets.
4. Place salmon on the prepared baking sheet.
5. Bake for 15-20 minutes, or until the salmon is cooked through and flakes easily with a fork.
6. While the salmon is baking, prepare the salsa. In a medium bowl, combine berries, red onion, lime juice, cilantro, and red pepper flakes (if using).
7. Serve the cooked salmon with a dollop of berry salsa on the side.

Nutritional Facts (per serving)

- Calories: 420
- Protein: 30g
- Fat: 22g (including healthy fats from salmon and olive oil)
- Carbohydrates: 25g
- Fiber: 4g

Tips

- Substitute other types of fish like cod or halibut for salmon.
- Choose your favorite berries for the salsa. Experiment with raspberries, blackberries, or a combination.

- For a milder salsa, omit the red pepper flakes.
- Leftovers can be stored in an airtight container in the refrigerator for up to 3 days.

One-Pan Lemon Garlic Shrimp with Leafy Greens

Ingredients

- 1 pound raw shrimp, peeled and deveined
- 1 tablespoon olive oil
- 2 cloves garlic, minced
- 1/2 teaspoon dried oregano
- 1/4 cup lemon juice
- 1/4 cup chicken broth (or vegetable broth)
- 4 cups baby spinach or mixed leafy greens
- Salt and freshly ground black pepper to taste

Instructions

1. Heat olive oil in a large skillet over medium heat.
2. Add shrimp and cook for 2-3 minutes per side, or until pink and opaque.
3. Stir in garlic and oregano, cook for 30 seconds, until fragrant.

4. Add lemon juice, chicken broth, salt, and pepper. Bring to a simmer and cook for 1-2 minutes, or until the sauce thickens slightly.
5. Add the leafy greens and toss with the shrimp and sauce until wilted.
6. Serve immediately and enjoy!

Nutritional Facts (per serving):

- Calories: 350
- Protein: 30g
- Fat: 15g (including healthy fats from olive oil)
- Carbohydrates: 10g
- Fiber: 2g

Tips:

- Use frozen, thawed shrimp for convenience.
- Experiment with different herbs like thyme or basil instead of oregano.
- To add a touch of heat, stir in a pinch of red pepper flakes with the garlic.
- Leftovers can be stored in an airtight container in the refrigerator for up to 1 day.

Vegetarian Chili with Quinoa and Black Beans

Ingredients

- 1 tablespoon olive oil
- 1 onion, chopped
- 1 green bell pepper, chopped
- 2 cloves garlic, minced
- 1 teaspoon chili powder
- 1/2 teaspoon cumin
- 1/4 teaspoon smoked paprika
- 1 (28-ounce) can crushed tomatoes
- 1 (15-ounce) can black beans, rinsed and drained
- 1 cup cooked quinoa
- 4 cups vegetable broth
- 1 cup frozen corn
- Salt and freshly ground black pepper to taste
- Optional toppings: chopped avocado, chopped fresh cilantro, shredded cheese (omit for a vegan option)

Instructions

1. Heat olive oil in a large pot or Dutch oven over medium heat.

2. Add onion, bell pepper, and garlic. Cook for 5-7 minutes, or until softened.
3. Stir in chili powder, cumin, and smoked paprika. Cook for an additional minute, allowing the spices to release their aroma.
4. Add crushed tomatoes, black beans, cooked quinoa, vegetable broth, and corn.
5. Bring to a boil, then reduce heat and simmer for 20-25 minutes, or until flavors have melded.
6. Season with salt and pepper to taste.
7. Serve hot, topped with desired toppings.

Nutritional Facts (per serving):

- Calories: 400
- Protein: 18g
- Fat: 12g (including healthy fats from olive oil)
- Carbohydrates: 55g
- Fiber: 10g

Tips:

- Feel free to add other vegetables to the chili, such as chopped carrots, zucchini, or mushrooms.
- Use pre-cooked quinoa for added convenience.

- To make the chili spicier, add a chopped jalapeno pepper with the onions and bell peppers.
- Leftovers can be stored in an airtight container in the refrigerator for up to 3 days.

Creamy Spinach and Mushroom Pasta with Walnuts

Ingredients

- 12 ounces whole-wheat pasta
- 1 tablespoon olive oil
- 1 onion, chopped
- 8 ounces mushrooms, sliced
- 2 cloves garlic, minced
- 1/4 cup chopped walnuts
- 1 cup low-fat milk (or unsweetened almond milk)
- 1 tablespoon cornstarch
- 1/4 cup grated Parmesan cheese
- 4 cups baby spinach
- Salt and freshly ground black pepper to taste

Instructions

1. Cook pasta according to package directions, reserving about 1/2 cup of the pasta water before draining.

2. While the pasta is cooking, heat olive oil in a large skillet over medium heat.
3. Add onion and cook for 5 minutes, or until softened.
4. Add mushrooms and cook for an additional 5 minutes, or until tender.
5. Stir in garlic and walnuts, cook for 30 seconds, until fragrant.
6. In a small bowl, whisk together milk and cornstarch to form a slurry.
7. Add the milk mixture and Parmesan cheese to the skillet with the cooked vegetables. Bring to a simmer and cook for 2-3 minutes, or until the sauce thickens slightly.
8. Stir in the spinach and cook until wilted.
9. Add the cooked pasta and reserved pasta water to the skillet. Toss to combine and coat the pasta in the sauce.
10. Season with salt and pepper to taste.
11. Serve immediately and enjoy!

Nutritional Facts (per serving):

- Calories: 500
- Protein: 20g
- Fat: 20g (including healthy fats from olive oil and walnuts)
- Carbohydrates: 60g

- Fiber: 5g

Tips:

- Use any type of whole-wheat pasta you like, such as penne, farfalle, or rotini.
- For a vegan option, omit the Parmesan cheese and use a vegan cheese alternative or nutritional yeast.
- To make the dish lighter, use low-fat ricotta cheese instead of the creamy sauce.
- Leftovers can be stored in an airtight container in the refrigerator for up to 2 days.

Baked Eggs with Frittata Toppings

This recipe offers a fun and customizable way to enjoy eggs for dinner. Bake eggs in individual ramekins with a variety of delicious toppings for a satisfying and protein-rich meal.

Ingredients:

- 4 eggs
- 1 tablespoon olive oil
- 1/4 cup chopped vegetables (such as bell peppers, onions, mushrooms)
- 1/4 cup crumbled feta cheese (optional)

- 1/4 cup chopped spinach
- Salt and freshly ground black pepper to taste
- Optional toppings: chopped fresh herbs, crumbled cooked sausage, shredded cheese

Instructions:

1. Preheat oven to 400°F (200°C). Lightly grease four ramekins.
2. Heat olive oil in a skillet over medium heat. Add chopped vegetables and cook for 5 minutes, or until softened.
3. Divide the cooked vegetables among the prepared ramekins.
4. Crack one egg into each ramekin. Season with salt and pepper.
5. Top each egg with desired toppings, such as crumbled feta cheese, chopped spinach, or cooked sausage.
6. Bake for 15-20 minutes, or until the egg whites are set and the yolks are cooked to your desired doneness.
7. Garnish with chopped fresh herbs (optional) and serve immediately.

Nutritional Facts (per serving, without feta cheese):

- Calories: 280

- Protein: 18g
- Fat: 15g (including healthy fats from olive oil)
- Carbohydrates: 5g
- Fiber: 1g

Tips:

- Experiment with different vegetable and topping combinations to create your own unique baked eggs.
- Use pre-cooked chopped vegetables for added convenience.
- Leftovers can be stored in an airtight container in the refrigerator for up to 1 day.

Salmon Burgers with Almond Flour Buns

These salmon burgers are a healthy and flavorful alternative to traditional beef burgers. Served on almond flour buns for a grain-free option, they are perfect for a satisfying and protein-packed dinner.

Ingredients

- For the salmon burgers:
- 1 pound salmon fillet, skin removed and flaked
- 1/4 cup chopped red onion
- 1/4 cup chopped fresh dill

- 1 egg, beaten
- 1/4 cup almond flour
- 1 tablespoon olive oil
- Salt and freshly ground black pepper to taste
- For the almond flour buns (makes 4 buns):
- 1/2 cup almond flour
- 1/4 cup ground flaxseed meal
- 1/4 teaspoon baking powder
- 1/4 teaspoon baking soda
- 1/4 cup unsweetened almond milk
- 1 tablespoon melted coconut oil
- 1 egg

Instructions:

1. Preheat oven to 400°F (200°C). Line a baking sheet with parchment paper.

For the salmon burgers:

2. In a large bowl, combine flaked salmon, red onion, dill, egg, almond flour, olive oil, salt, and pepper. Mix well to combine.
3. Form the salmon mixture into four equal patties.
4. Place the salmon patties on the prepared baking sheet.

5. Bake for 15-20 minutes, or until cooked through and golden brown.

For the almond flour buns:

1. In a medium bowl, whisk together almond flour, flaxseed meal, baking powder, and baking soda.
2. In a separate bowl, whisk together almond milk, melted coconut oil, and egg.
3. Pour the wet ingredients into the dry ingredients and mix until just combined. Avoid overmixing.
4. Divide the batter evenly among four greased ramekins or muffin tins.
5. Bake for 20-25 minutes, or until the buns are golden brown and a toothpick inserted into the center comes out clean.

Assembly:

6. Once the salmon patties and buns are cooked, assemble the burgers.
7. Toast the buns slightly, if desired.
8. Place a salmon patty on each bun bottom.
9. Add your favorite burger toppings, such as lettuce, tomato, sliced avocado, or a light drizzle of your favorite sauce.
10. Top with the bun top and enjoy!

Nutritional Facts (per serving, with almond flour buns):

- Calories: 500
- Protein: 40g
- Fat: 30g (including healthy fats from salmon and coconut oil)
- Carbohydrates: 15g
- Fiber: 5g

Tips:

- You can grill the salmon patties instead of baking them for a smoky flavor.
- If the salmon mixture seems too wet, add a little more almond flour until it holds its shape.
- For a vegan option, use a flaxseed egg instead of a regular egg in both the salmon burgers and the buns.
- Leftover salmon patties can be stored in an airtight container in the refrigerator for up to 2 days.

Chicken Stir-Fry with Vegetables and Brown Rice

Ingredients

- 1 pound boneless, skinless chicken breasts, cut into bite-sized pieces

- 1 tablespoon olive oil
- 1 onion, sliced
- 1 bell pepper, sliced
- 1 cup broccoli florets
- 1/2 cup sugar snap peas
- 2 cloves garlic, minced
- 1 tablespoon soy sauce
- 1 tablespoon rice vinegar
- 1 tablespoon cornstarch
- 1/4 cup water
- 2 cups cooked brown rice
- Salt and freshly ground black pepper to taste

Instructions:

- In a small bowl, whisk together soy sauce, rice vinegar, cornstarch, and water. Set aside.
- Heat olive oil in a large skillet or wok over medium-high heat.
- Add chicken pieces and cook for 5-7 minutes, or until golden brown and cooked through. Remove the chicken from the pan and set aside.

- Add onion, bell pepper, broccoli florets, and sugar snap peas to the pan. Stir-fry for 5-7 minutes, or until the vegetables are tender-crisp.
- Add the minced garlic and cook for an additional 30 seconds, until fragrant.
- Pour the soy sauce mixture into the pan and bring to a simmer. Cook for 1-2 minutes, or until the sauce thickens slightly.
- Add the cooked chicken back to the pan and toss to coat in the sauce.
- Serve the stir-fry over cooked brown rice and enjoy!

Nutritional Facts (per serving):

- Calories: 450
- Protein: 35g
- Fat: 15g (including healthy fats from olive oil)
- Carbohydrates: 40g
- Fiber: 5g

Tips:

- Feel free to use other vegetables in the stir-fry, such as carrots, mushrooms, or baby corn.

- Serve the stir-fry with a sprinkle of sesame seeds or chopped peanuts for added flavor and texture.
- Leftovers can be stored in an airtight container in the refrigerator for up to 3 days.

Lentil Soup with Leafy Greens and Lemon

Ingredients:

- 1 tablespoon olive oil
- 1 onion, chopped
- 2 cloves garlic, minced
- 1 teaspoon dried thyme
- 1 cup brown lentils, rinsed
- 4 cups vegetable broth
- 4 cups chopped kale or spinach
- 1 lemon, juiced
- Salt and freshly ground black pepper to taste

Instructions

1. Heat olive oil in a large pot or Dutch oven over medium heat.
2. Add onion and cook for 5 minutes, or until softened.
3. Stir in garlic and thyme, cook for 30 seconds, until fragrant.

4. Add lentils and vegetable broth. Bring to a boil, then reduce heat and simmer for 20-25 minutes, or until lentils are tender.
5. Add the chopped kale or spinach and cook for an additional 2-3 minutes, or until wilted.
6. Stir in lemon juice and season with salt and pepper to taste.
7. Serve hot and enjoy!

Nutritional Facts (per serving)

- Calories: 300
- Protein: 15g
- Fat: 10g (including healthy fats from olive oil)
- Carbohydrates: 40g
- Fiber: 10g

Tips

- Use pre-cooked lentils for added convenience.
- To make the soup creamier, blend a portion of the cooked soup with an immersion blender before adding it back to the pot.
- Leftovers can be stored in an airtight container in the refrigerator for up to 3 days.

Vegetarian Stuffed Peppers

Ingredients

- 4 bell peppers, any color
- 1 tablespoon olive oil
- 1 onion, chopped
- 1 clove garlic, minced
- 1 cup cooked brown rice
- 1/2 cup cooked quinoa
- 1 cup chopped zucchini
- 1/2 cup chopped mushrooms
- 1 (15-ounce) can black beans, rinsed and drained
- 1/2 cup chopped fresh parsley
- 1/4 cup chopped fresh cilantro
- 1/4 cup grated Parmesan cheese (optional)
- Salt and freshly ground black pepper to taste

Instructions

1. Preheat oven to 400°F (200°C).
2. Cut the tops off the bell peppers and remove the seeds and membranes. Rinse the peppers and pat them dry.
3. Heat olive oil in a large skillet over medium heat.
4. Add onion and cook for 5 minutes, or until softened.

5. Stir in garlic and cook for an additional 30 seconds, until fragrant.
6. Add cooked brown rice, quinoa, zucchini, mushrooms, black beans, parsley, and cilantro. Season with salt and pepper to taste. Cook for an additional 5 minutes, or until heated through.
7. Stuff the bell pepper halves with the vegetable mixture. Sprinkle with Parmesan cheese (if using).
8. Place the stuffed peppers in a baking dish and bake for 20-25 minutes, or until the peppers are tender and the filling is heated through.
9. Serve hot and enjoy!

Nutritional Facts (per serving, without Parmesan cheese):

- Calories: 400
- Protein: 18g
- Fat: 12g (including healthy fats from olive oil)
- Carbohydrates: 55g
- Fiber: 10g

Tips

- Use a variety of colored bell peppers for added visual appeal.

- You can pre-cook the bell peppers in the oven for 10 minutes before stuffing them to soften them slightly.
- Leftovers can be stored in an airtight container in the refrigerator for up to 3 days.

Tofu Scramble with Spinach and Tomatoes

Ingredients

- 1 block firm tofu, drained and pressed
- 1 tablespoon olive oil
- 1/2 onion, chopped
- 2 cloves garlic, minced
- 1/4 teaspoon turmeric powder
- 1/4 teaspoon smoked paprika
- 1/4 teaspoon black pepper
- 1 cup chopped spinach
- 1/2 cup chopped tomatoes
- 1/4 cup chopped fresh parsley
- Salt to taste
- Optional toppings: chopped avocado, nutritional yeast, hot sauce

Instructions

1. Crumble the tofu with your hands or a fork into a bowl.

2. Heat olive oil in a large skillet over medium heat.
3. Add onion and cook for 5 minutes, or until softened.
4. Stir in garlic, turmeric powder, smoked paprika, and black pepper. Cook for an additional 30 seconds, until fragrant.
5. Add the crumbled tofu to the pan and cook for 5-7 minutes, stirring occasionally, until slightly browned and crispy.
6. Add the chopped spinach and cook for an additional 2-3 minutes, or until wilted.
7. Stir in the chopped tomatoes and cook for another minute, or until heated through.
8. Season with salt to taste.
9. Remove from heat and stir in the chopped fresh parsley.
10. Serve immediately with your desired toppings, such as chopped avocado, nutritional yeast, or hot sauce.

Nutritional Facts (per serving)

- Calories: 300
- Protein: 20g
- Fat: 15g (including healthy fats from olive oil)
- Carbohydrates: 20g
- Fiber: 5g

Tips

- To press the tofu, wrap it in a clean kitchen towel and place a heavy object on top for 15-20 minutes. This will remove excess moisture and allow the tofu to crumble more easily.
- Feel free to add other vegetables to the scramble, such as chopped mushrooms, bell peppers, or onions.
- Leftovers can be stored in an airtight container in the refrigerator for up to 2 days.

Chicken and Vegetable Curry with Coconut Milk
Ingredients

- 1 tablespoon olive oil
- 1 onion, chopped
- 2 cloves garlic, minced
- 1 tablespoon curry powder
- 1 teaspoon ground ginger
- 1/2 teaspoon turmeric powder
- 1 (13.5-ounce) can coconut milk
- 1 pound boneless, skinless chicken breasts, cut into bite-sized pieces
- 1 cup chopped bell peppers (any color)
- 1 cup chopped broccoli florets
- 1/2 cup chopped carrots

- 1 cup chopped tomatoes
- 1 cup cooked brown rice
- Salt and freshly ground black pepper to taste
- Optional toppings: chopped fresh cilantro, chopped peanuts

Instructions

1. Heat olive oil in a large pot or Dutch oven over medium heat.
2. Add onion and cook for 5 minutes, or until softened.
3. Stir in garlic, curry powder, ginger, and turmeric powder. Cook for an additional 30 seconds, until fragrant.
4. Add the coconut milk and bring to a simmer.
5. Add the chicken pieces and cook for 5-7 minutes, or until golden brown and cooked through.
6. Add the chopped bell peppers, broccoli florets, carrots, and tomatoes. Simmer for an additional 10-15 minutes, or until the vegetables are tender-crisp.
7. Stir in the cooked brown rice and season with salt and pepper to taste.
8. Serve hot, topped with chopped fresh cilantro and chopped peanuts (if using).

Nutritional Facts (per serving):

- Calories: 500
- Protein: 40g
- Fat: 20g (including healthy fats from coconut milk)
- Carbohydrates: 40g
- Fiber: 5g

Tips:

- You can use other vegetables in the curry, such as green beans, zucchini, or eggplant.
- Adjust the curry powder to your desired level of spiciness.
- Leftovers can be stored in an airtight container in the refrigerator for up to 3 days.

One-Pan Roasted Chicken with Root Vegetables

Ingredients

- 1 whole chicken (around 3-4 pounds)
- 1 tablespoon olive oil
- 1/2 teaspoon dried thyme
- 1/2 teaspoon paprika
- Salt and freshly ground black pepper to taste

- 4 medium potatoes, peeled and cut into wedges
- 2 carrots, peeled and cut into chunks
- 1 onion, cut into wedges
- 2 cloves garlic, minced

Instructions

1. Preheat oven to 400°F (200°C).
2. Pat the chicken dry with paper towels. Season the cavity and skin generously with olive oil, thyme, paprika, salt, and pepper.
3. In a large roasting pan, toss the potatoes, carrots, and onion with olive oil, salt, and pepper.
4. Place the chicken on top of the vegetables. Scatter the garlic cloves around the pan.
5. Roast for 1-1/2 to 2 hours, or until the chicken is cooked through and the vegetables are tender. The internal temperature of the chicken thigh should reach 165°F (74°C).
6. Let the chicken rest for 10 minutes before carving and serving with the roasted vegetables.

Nutritional Facts (per serving):

- Calories: 500

- Protein: 45g
- Fat: 25g (including healthy fats from olive oil)
- Carbohydrates: 40g
- Fiber: 5g

Tips:

- You can add other root vegetables to the roasting pan, such as parsnips, turnips, or beets.
- Stuff the chicken cavity with chopped lemons, oranges, or herbs for additional flavor.
- Leftovers can be stored in an airtight container in the refrigerator for up to 3 days.

Turkey Burgers with Sweet Potato Fries

Ingredients

- For the turkey burgers:
- 1 pound ground turkey
- 1/4 cup chopped onion
- 1/4 cup chopped fresh parsley
- 1 egg, beaten
- 1/4 cup breadcrumbs
- 1 tablespoon olive oil

- Salt and freshly ground black pepper to taste
- For the sweet potato fries:
- 2 large sweet potatoes, peeled and cut into wedges
- 1 tablespoon olive oil
- 1/2 teaspoon paprika
- Salt and freshly ground black pepper to taste

Instructions

1. Preheat oven to 400°F (200°C).
2. In a large bowl, combine ground turkey, chopped onion, parsley, egg, breadcrumbs, olive oil, salt, and pepper. Mix well to combine.
3. Form the turkey mixture into four equal patties.
4. Heat a large skillet over medium heat. Add a drizzle of olive oil and cook the turkey burgers for 5-7 minutes per side, or until cooked through.

For the sweet potato fries:

5. Toss the sweet potato wedges with olive oil, paprika, salt, and pepper.
6. Spread the sweet potato wedges on a baking sheet in a single layer.

7. Bake for 20-25 minutes, or until tender-crisp and golden brown, flipping halfway through cooking.

Assembly:

8. Serve the turkey burgers on hamburger buns with your desired toppings, such as lettuce, tomato, sliced avocado, or your favorite sauce.
9. Enjoy alongside the crispy sweet potato fries.

Nutritional Facts (per serving):

- Calories: 550
- Protein: 40g
- Fat: 25g (including healthy fats from olive oil)
- Carbohydrates: 50g
- Fiber: 10g

Tips

- You can grill the turkey burgers instead of cooking them in a skillet.
- For a vegan option, use a plant-based burger patty instead of ground turkey.
- Leftover burgers can be stored in an airtight container in the refrigerator for up to 2 days.

Lentil and Vegetable Shepherd's Pie

Chicken and Quinoa Stuffed Peppers

Ingredients

- 4 bell peppers (any color)
- 1 tablespoon olive oil
- 1 onion, chopped
- 1 clove garlic, minced
- 1 pound ground chicken
- 1 cup cooked quinoa
- 1/2 cup chopped zucchini
- 1/2 cup chopped mushrooms
- 1/4 cup chopped fresh parsley
- 1 (14.5-ounce) can diced tomatoes, undrained
- 1 teaspoon chili powder
- 1/2 teaspoon cumin
- Salt and freshly ground black pepper to taste
- 1/4 cup shredded cheddar cheese (optional)

Instructions

1. Preheat oven to 400°F (200°C).
2. Cut the tops off the bell peppers and remove the seeds and membranes. Rinse the peppers and pat them dry.

3. Heat olive oil in a large skillet over medium heat.
4. Add onion and cook for 5 minutes, or until softened.
5. Stir in garlic and cook for an additional 30 seconds, until fragrant.
6. Add ground chicken and cook, breaking it up with a spoon, until browned.
7. Drain any excess grease from the pan.
8. Stir in cooked quinoa, chopped zucchini, mushrooms, chopped parsley, diced tomatoes, chili powder, cumin, salt, and pepper.
9. Simmer for 5 minutes, or until heated through.

Assembly:

10. Spoon the chicken and quinoa mixture into the prepared bell pepper halves.
11. Sprinkle with shredded cheddar cheese (if using).
12. Place the stuffed peppers in a baking dish and bake for 20-25 minutes, or until the peppers are tender and the filling is heated through.

Nutritional Facts (per serving, without cheese):

- Calories: 450
- Protein: 35g

- Fat: 18g (including healthy fats from olive oil)
- Carbohydrates: 40g
- Fiber: 5g

Tips

- You can use other vegetables in the stuffing, such as chopped carrots, peas, or corn.
- For a vegetarian option, omit the ground chicken and add an extra cup of cooked quinoa.
- Leftovers can be stored in an airtight container in the refrigerator for up to 3 days.

Salmon with Roasted Vegetables and Lemon Dill Sauce

Ingredients:

- 4 salmon fillets (around 6 ounces each)
- 1 tablespoon olive oil
- Salt and freshly ground black pepper to taste
- For the roasted vegetables:
- 1 head of broccoli, cut into florets
- 1 red bell pepper, sliced
- 1 yellow squash, sliced
- 1 zucchini, sliced

- 1 tablespoon olive oil
- 1/2 teaspoon dried thyme
- Salt and freshly ground black pepper to taste
- For the lemon dill sauce:
- 1/4 cup low-fat yogurt (or sour cream)
- 1 tablespoon freshly squeezed lemon juice
- 1 tablespoon chopped fresh dill
- Salt and freshly ground black pepper to taste

Instructions

1. Preheat oven to 400°F (200°C). Line a baking sheet with parchment paper.
2. Toss the broccoli florets, bell pepper slices, yellow squash slices, and zucchini slices with olive oil, thyme, salt, and pepper.
3. Spread the vegetables on the prepared baking sheet and roast for 15-20 minutes, or until tender-crisp.
4. **For the salmon:**
5. Pat the salmon fillets dry with paper towels. Season with olive oil, salt, and pepper.
6. Place the salmon fillets on a separate baking sheet.

For the lemon dill sauce:

7. In a small bowl, whisk together yogurt (or sour cream), lemon juice, chopped dill, salt, and pepper.

Assembly:

8. Bake the salmon for 12-15 minutes, or until cooked through and flakes easily with a fork.
9. Serve the salmon over the roasted vegetables and top with the lemon dill sauce.

Nutritional Facts (per serving):

- Calories: 450
- Protein: 30g
- Fat: 20g

CONCLUSION

Living with Polymyalgia Rheumatica can be challenging, but you don't have to navigate it alone. This comprehensive guide empowers you to take control of your health through the power of food. By incorporating delicious and anti-inflammatory recipes into your diet, you can experience symptom relief, boost your energy levels, and promote overall well-being. Remember, a healthy diet is just one piece of the puzzle. This book also provides valuable tips for exercise, sleep, stress management, and building a strong support system. With a proactive approach and a positive outlook, you can manage Polymyalgia Rheumatica and live a fulfilling life.

Printed in Great Britain
by Amazon